RINGWORM

RINGWORM
ITS CONSTITUTIONAL NATURE AND CURE

By

J. Compton Burnett M.D.

GYAN

Published by

GYAN

Gyan Publishing House
5, Ansari Road
Daryaganj, New Delhi-110002
Phone: 011-47034999, 9811692060
E-mail: books@gyanbooks.com

Distribution Network
gyanbooks.com
India, USA, Canada, UK, Australia, France

ISBN : 978-81-212-6601-7 (PB)
First Published, 1892

2nd Impression 2022

Printed at: Gyan Press, Delhi.

RINGWORM: ITS CONSTITUTIONAL NATURE AND CURE
Author: J. COMPTON BURNETT

RINGWORM:

ITS CONSTITUTIONAL NATURE AND CURE.

BY

J. COMPTON BURNETT, M.D.

Il faut, pour la réalisation de la maladie, la réunion de deux facteurs; le premier nécessaire, est le germe infectieux, le second, non moins indispensable, est la connivence de l'organisme qui mettra à la disposition du germe l'ensemble des conditions physiques et chimiques qui constituent son milieu vivant. A cette condition, et à cette condition seulement, la maladie sera constituée.—BOUCHARD (*Les Microbes Pathogenes*).

PREFACE.

SOME years since I published a small volume under the title of *Diseases of the Skin from the Organismic Standpoint*, and in it I seek to show that the so-called diseases of the skin are for the most part diseases of the constitutions of the persons, and not diseases of their skins. Since that time I have had ample opportunities of making observations on the true nature of skin diseases, and these observations tend almost uniformly to prove the correctness of the view.

Gout in the big toe is not a disease of the said toe; acne on the shoulders of young persons is not a disease of the skin of the shoulders; neither is a yellow-coated tongue a disease of the tongue.

The disease under consideration in this tiny treatise is one of the most characteristic, and its outward nature is indisputably parasitic; yet a careful survey of the young individuals that get it shows that they all have very peculiar characteristics—ætiological, cutaneous, and glandular.

Ringworm inspires disgust; more or less almost all skin diseases do that, and yet a perfectly clear skin may enclose a very diseased organism, and a skin-diseased person may have a relatively much better constitution, and have all his internal organs in a relatively much better state, his cutaneous manifestations notwithstanding.

Indeed, I would almost go so far as to say that many cutaneous manifestations betoken, in a certain sense, constitutional power,—in the sense, namely, that such organism has the power to determine its diseases to the periphery, to its outside. It other words, the disease being of the organism, it is a smaller evil to have it outside on the skin than to have it inside in a given organ. Gouty inflammation of the big toe is one thing; the same process in the stomach, quite another; therefore, the disease being given, it is the stronger person who throws said disease *into* his skin; but that does not make it a disease *of* the skin. Old physicians who used to set up issues in their patients' flesh, and maintain them there, knew well what they were about.

In regard to ringworm I am of opinion that absolutely healthy children do not and cannot, catch it. Before they can catch ringworm it is essential that they be in tainted health in some way, for otherwise they could not supply to the parasitic fungi the food which they need to live and thrive on, and to continue their propagation. On careful reflection, this I believe will have to be conceded, and this the following pages illustrate clinically.

You cannot grow a common mushroom except under given conditions, neither can you the trichophyton of ringworm.

The trichophyton is not the disease itself, but its organic scavenger. Cure the internal disease, and this scavenger dies.

J. COMPTON BURNETT.

86 WIMPOLE STREET,
CAVANDISH SQUARE, W.,
August, 1892

RINGWORM:

HERPES S. TINEA TONSURANS.

THAT Ringworm (Herpes s. tinea tonsurans) is due to a specific fungus is one of the certainties of practical medicine; that the recognised treatment of the same is by external applications with the view of killing the fungi, no one needs to be told. Hitherto its medicability by internal remedies has been admitted by a certain section of the homœopathic school of medicine. Indeed the more staunch Hahnemannians have always fought for this view, and time and again have proved its practicability; on this point I have long been at one with these more staunch of the Hahnemannians, and that simply because I have been able to verify their views clinically. For years, in common with many others, I have been constantly in the habit of treating and curing ringworm by internal remedies with relative success. For all that I have thus far never had anything approaching to a clear notion of its true nature, and some of the cases would persist in not getting well; and this lack of a definite idea of its nature, and also the uncertainty of its cure, is I believe fully shared by those who have thus habitually considered and treated ringworm constitutionally. It is due, let us say, to psora, but we have no clear conception of what psora is. Psora needs to be split up into its component parts, no easy task; it roots in the vague, its trunk and boughs run away into anywhere. The psora of the homœopaths seems somehow true, but it has no proper beginning, no definite course, and ends in pathological chaos. Perhaps we study it in Hahnemann, and in the best writers on the subject, and after doing our best to master it, we rise from our studies with no clear idea, and we finally decide to abandon psora as an intangible myth, and then we proceed with our clinical work; but, before long, we stumble against a very tangible something, and on looking at the stumbling block, we find writ large upon it the word *Psora!* Have I then hit upon a solution of the psora-problem? No; but if we cannot break the whole faggot, we may perchance break one stick of it.

Hughes, in his *Manual of Therapeutics*, says that Herpes circinnatus (ringworm of the surface) is usually treated, and with fair success, by *Sepia*, but that when the proving of *Tellurium* produced so similar an eruption, he (Dr. Hughes) followed Dr. Metcalf in prescribing it instead of *Sepia* for this disorder, and has never failed to cure it speedily thereby.

Of ringworm proper of the

scalp, Hughes thus writes:—(*Manual of Therapeutics*, p. 520) "That this disease is, when recent, amenable to internal remedies alone seems to disprove the theory of its parasitic origin. The medicine for it is *Sepia*, at about the 6th dilution; but if this fails, you must resort to some local parasiticide, of which I suppose a solution of *Sulphurous acid* would be about the best."

Some time since I published a small volume, entitled *Five Years' Experience in the New Cure of Consumption by its own Virus*, and the fifty-third illustrative case therein runs thus (p. 95):—

The influence of the virus upon the teeth and their growth and appearance is very striking. What

I regard as tubercular teeth are those—often more or less rudimentary—with holes in their external surface. Whether this is a recognised pathological fact I do not happen to know, perhaps is it not. But it is an important clinical observation. I recognized it clinically some three years since, while treating a highly strumous lady with many scars and glands in her neck. While under the virus I noticed an extraordinary improvement in her teeth, they became a nice color, and the numerous superficial holes cleaned and partially disappeared. It was even more apparent and striking in the following case :—A girl of 11, with ringworm on the scalp ; the lymphatic glands everywhere palpable, and her ribs very flat; strawberry tongue; a bad cough, worse at night; although 11 years old she had practically no teeth, that is to say, they were rudimentary and not above the level of her gums. *All* her mother's brothers and sisters had died of consumption; after three months' treatment with our ordinary remedies we had made but small progress, and then I kept patient altogether five month under the bacillic virus, with the result that her palpable glans ceased to be palpable; her ringworm disappeared; her ribs took on a better form; her breathing was notably better; and, *mirabile dictu, her teeth had grown.* She is now well, and has a mouthful of teeth which are quite passible. It may be noted that the ringworm had disappeared, and in respect to this nasty thing I find it generally disappears under the influence of the virus. I learned this very important fact also purely clinically in the following manner: —A whole family of children of different ages had had ringworm for a full year, and the mother told me on bringing them that she had already spent over £60 on medical fees for its cure, but in vain. All known remedies had been applied by the local doctors in two neighbourhoods, and several skin specialists had worked hard at their poor heads, but to no avail. Their heads were shaved and their scalps were well scoured night and morning but *still* the ringworm persisted. Finally, a distant cottage had been hired, and the afflicted ones were there isolated, and the services of a noted ringworm curer of the non-qualified variety had been secured; but these also failing, they were put under my care. I have had no great cause to complain of the homœopathic treatment of ringworm with our antipsorics—indeed, quite the contrary—but it is apt to be a bit tedious at times. Now their mother had been cured by me of incipient tuberculosis with the virus, and it occurred to me that ringworm might be a manifestation of the tubercular kind,* and so I forthwith put the whole lot under the virus, administered in the usual way, internally in dynamic dose; this I

* I find Tilbury Fox and Startin were of this opinion; so are, doubtless, many others.

did all the more readily, as they all had numerous superficial palpable glands. And the result? In a very few weeks they were all well of ringworm and of the glands, and have thriven splendidly ever since. Something like a dozen bad ringworm cases have come to me since then, and they were *all* quickly cured by the virus, and in each case the general state has been greatly improved. No doubt some bacteriologists will cultivate, some fine day, the germs of the ringworm; and astound the world with their subcutaneous injections. It is well that medical men should approach each subject from a different standpoint, as they serve to correct one another.

Since then I have systematically

subjected almost all my ringworm cases to the influence of Bacillinum in high potency and infrequently administered, and of this later experience I will now proceed to treat. Ringworm is a fairly common complaint, and sends terror into the hearts of masters and mistresses of houses; and schoolmasters and school mistresses give but a short shrift to any unfortunate wights who show on their scalps or necks, or elsewhere, anything approaching to a scaly, ring-like patch. They know well that if it spreads, or is reported to the children's homes, the depletion of their school is imminent. "No Doctor; I am very fond of Gerald, he is my own nephew, and a dear good boy, and his father is in India, but I cannot take him back to my school unless you give me a written certificate, *and that round patch on his neck is quite cured!*" The very Prince of Darkness is less dreaded in a school than ringworm. Definite information, therefore, on the subject of the nature *and cure* of ringworm will be welcome to not a few. Moreover, it marks a new era in the treatment of the disease. When I say it marks a new era in the treatment of the disease, I should say that for the first time it gives us a clue to its ætiology, pathology, and, best of all, to its really radical cure. The metamorphosis wrought in the bad or poor constitutions of ringworm patients subjected to the influence of Bacillinum (high, and mark well, in very infrequent doses) is simply beautiful, and a delight to the heart of the physician who loves his work for its own sake, and the more so if he has a fair share of the milk of human kindness in him.

I do not agree with those who consider that the amenability of ringworm to internal treatment—say to *Sulphur*, *Sepia*, *or Tellurium* — militates against its parasitic nature.* There can be no question of its parasitic nature, however it may be cured. We must read the facts thus: the disease *is* parasitic in its external manifestation, and if this external manifestation—the scaly, annular patches — be the

* I think Erasmus Wilson could never be brought to believe in the parasitic nature of ringworm.

disease, and the whole of the disease, then, of course, internal treatment must be regarded as little less than silly, and the only sensible thing to do is to apply to the ringworm parts something that shall kill the fungi and therefore cure the disease.

Well, few need to be told that the task of treating ringworm successfully by external means, *i.e.*, killing the fungi, is so unsatisfactory, so uncertain, so tedious, so often an entire failure, that I well understand the state of mind of an eminent London skin specialist, who six weeks ago exclaimed to Lady X., who wished to known *how long* it would be before her little boy would be quite cured of his ringworm, and fit to return to school, "How long? Heaven knows, I don't; perhaps by the end of next term, I really cannot say!"

And thus it is: the external treatment of ringworm is wrong, because it only deals with the external manifestations of the internal organismic ailment. RINGWORM IS AN INTERNAL DISEASE *of the organism having for its outward sign the ringworm consisting of fungi thriving in a certain order:* the fungi are the guests of the diseased host; cure the host's diseased state, and the fungus—the ringworm—dies off from lack of a proper medium. Ringworm may be regarded as mould of the skin, analogous to the mould on cheese, bits of bread, oranges, or lemons, and warm moisture favours its development. Mouldy products love darkness rather than light—a sort of half light, moisture, warmth, and hiddenness; decaying organic matter is their food and life, and I am satisfied that those who get ringworm have in their scalps something whereon the ringworm mould can live, thrive, and multiply.

Inveterate Case of Herpes Tonsurans, or Ringworm.

A lad of eight years of age was brought to me at the end of April 1891, to be treated for ringworm, under a very severe form of which he had been labouring for over a year. At the date in question it was nearly all over his body, scalp, neck, upper extremities, in large numbers of rings, varying in size from that of a sixpenny piece to that of a halfpenny. His scalp is one mass of scabs and scales extending all down his neck (said to have come from goapowder). The scalp is at times moist. He has no feelable glands in his neck, but those of his groins are like so many very small marbles. Sparsely strawberry-like tongue; teeth yellow and decaying.

"What have you tried for your son?"

"Tried! everything, but he gets worse and worse, and since that goapowder his head has gone like that."

I am sure that any experienced practitioner of medicine, who places his faith in the outside treatment of ringworm, recognises the picture

I am drawing as that of a type of ringworm cases that *will not* get well do what we will. I have had them myself in olden days, till I hated the very sight of them, with their closely shaven scalps that seemed to consist in a number of little exits of sticky, mattery ooze that then dried into scabs. Such was this boy's aspect, but some of its hideousness was covered by a natty, well-fitting skull-cap.

Bacillinum C. was given for two months, when on the 24th June, I find noted that the red pips of his tongue were nearly gone; the lower half of his scalp was clean and healthy; appetite better; teeth much cleaner and whiter. "He is much better in his health."

To continue with the same remedy.

July 29th, 1891.—He is quite well of his ringworm, though his scalp is slightly scurfy, and his teeth still rather dirty looking. He then had the same remedy (1000th), whereafter the only one thing wrong with him was the greeny state of his teeth, which presumably was from another ætiological source, and therefore not amenable to the bacillinic influence. A worse case of ringworm would, indeed, be hard to find: a prettier, cleaner, or more accurately scientific cure I do not ask for. When cured the boy was a picture, with his splendid crop of hair stubbles about an inch in length—and, moreover, in excellent general health.

I used *no* external remedies at all. I do not for one moment suppose that the medical world (and still less the surgical) will accept my statements in regard to the true nature and cure of ringworm; nor do I imagine that they will fairly try my treatment. Past experience teaches me, that really radical curing on lines of scientific precision with high homœopathic potencies is not in harmony with prevailing views, and, therefore, totally incomprehensible and unacceptable to the profession at large, and hardly more acceptable to eight-tenths of the medical men practising homœopathically. Even the homœopathic practitioner seems very commonly quite unable to crawl out of his own old ways. Well, medical progress will pass him by and go on.

The internal treatment of ringworm by *Sulphur*, *Sepia*, and *Tellurium* is good, but I trust I shall be able in these pages to show that the treatment of ringworm by the internal administration of very infrequent doses of high potencies of *Bacillinum* is direct, exact, radical, and beyond compare; the remedy being pathologically homœopathic to the whole morbid state and crasis of the individual, and not merely pathologically similar to the superficial cutaneous manifestations.

I have long maintained the organismic or constitutional nature of skin diseases, and have time and again defended the thesis in medical literature, notably in my small treatise, *Diseases of the Skin from the Organismic Stand-point*, which is here confirmed in a manner I had not even hoped for, viz., direct clinical proof of the thesis that skin diseases are indeed general, constitutional, or organismic; and, therefore, for very joy I will dwell upon ringworm pretty fully, for as I have discovered that it is curable by the administration of *Bacillinum* in high potency, it so comes to pass that I can demonstrate clinically the organismic nature and cure of an affection of the skin that is clearly outside, to all intents and purposes, in its own life-history, being admittedly and demonstrably due to the fungus known as the trichophyton. And this demonstration is all the more powerful, because we cannot deny that the herpes tonsurans, or ringworm, is due to this fungus, the trichophyton. No; we cannot, of course, since the thing is scientifically demonstrable, as Köbner inoculated himself and certain animals with its products, and ringworm was the result.

Ringworm is, therefore, an external disease due to an external infection, the trichophyton, and (next to the itch) *the* skin disease of which people have the very greatest horror. This is due, in the first place, to the fact that its favourite seat is the hairy scalp, or near it, though we find it often in other parts of the body, and it causes the hair to fall out in circular patches as if eaten away in a ring by little worms, and hence our

English name of ringworm. Therefore, any lady's imagination readily paints herself to herself with any number of these round "spots" with loss of hair, and thus an object to be shunned,—and ladies do not, as a rule, wish to be shunned. Next to this horror is the disgrace(!) of being subject to such a disgusting disease; and, finally, it is very well known to be often exceedingly difficult of cure.

"Oh, I have tried all our big doctors and two quacks, and all the sure cures, but M's head is worse than ever!" But all these trials were on the same lines, viz., external applications to kill the fungi.

What first struck me was the fact, that in a given household infected by ringworm only *some* of the members got the disease, and these were invariably the weaker ones, the weedy, and the unhealthy. I have known households in which ringworm existed in one or two of its members, and although towels, brushes and combs were used almost indiscriminately, still the disease did *not* spread. Conversely I have known others in which only one child would have, perhaps, just one small patch, and in which the greatest care was taken to prevent the thing spreading, yet many of the children finally caught the complaint

I have noticed the same with cattle. Thus, a herd of heifers of my own observing two years ago, numbering eighteen when mustered in the yard, were examined by me for ringworm, and five had it—three pretty badly. These five were relatively weedy specimens, and those that had it worse were the most weedy. I noticed that the infected ones rubbed the diseased parts against posts and the like, and the healthy ones living with them, grazing in the same meadows, eating out of the same bins, herded with them in the same yard at night, all rubbing against one another, and against the same hard objects. The healthy ones, I saw, remained healthy and *did not* take ringworm in the smallest degree.

A practical cattle-kenner standing by was questioned by me as to this ringworm. "Oh," said he, "the healthy, strong ones will *not* get it."

"And what do you do to cure the diseased ones?" "Oh, that's nothing; keep them dry, litter the yard well, feed them well, and they will all get well of the ringworm *as soon as they get strong.*"

I took particular notice of this herd for many months, and found, indeed, that the ringwormy ones mended of their ringworm exactly in proportion to their general improvement, and in the end only one remained unimproved, and that one had always been the most weedy, and it was thought that she would die. I had no further opportunity of observing the herd, but I had seen quite enough to satisfy myself that strong, healthy heifers do not get ringworm although exposed to the infection closely and constantly, and those that have it get rid of it in direct proportion to the improvement in their general condition. In other words, the ringworm fungi cannot live and thrive in really healthy animals, and the ill condition of those that have the disease is not a consequence of the disease, but a necessary antecedent condition of the animals before the trichophyton can thrive.

Whether ringworm in itself is beneficial or hurtful, I am unable to say with certainty, but incline strongly to the belief that it may be beneficial. When I say that I incline strongly to the belief that it may be beneficial, I mean that the presence of the fungi being sequential to internal ill-conditionedness, and being on the outside of the economy, may live on what harms that individual, and thus determine the hurtful matter from the within to the outside, thus acting as living derivatives.

Inquiring of my practical cattle-kenner whether the men who tend ringwormy cattle catch the disease or not, he said,—"Oh, yes, sometimes, but not as a rule."

The man who attended to this particular herd of heifers did catch the disease; and I found on examining him that he was phthisically disposed, he was very dusky, he tanned unduly in the sun, was morose and taciturn, and always felt tired and weary. I found, further, that he had had to give up a good situation in a large town, and had been recommended to find an outdoor occupation in the country, the doctors telling him he would go into consumption if he stayed in the town.

I remember years ago attending the family of a farmer, when several of the children were presented to me as having caught ringworm from the cows, and one of the boys afterwards became very distinctly consumptive, and was given up as past praying for, and then he was sent up to London to me. Four months of *Bacillinum*, high, quite cured him, and he is now thriving.

This all confirms me in my view, which is the underlying idea of this book, that there is some close relationship between tuberculosis and ringworm, the precise nature of which deserves attention and study.

I have already quoted from the first London edition of my *Five Years' Experience in the New Cure of Consumption*, which see.

In the second (American) edition of this same work the following may be found:—

Case of Ringworm.

In the first edition, as just stated, I communicated the important fact —many smaller things are called great discoveries—that ringworm yields readily to *Bacillinum*, and that I therefore regard this cutaneous eruption as a tubercular manifestation. A little girl, five and a half years of age, was brought to me at the end of January 1891 to be treated for ringworm; there was only one ring on the back of the neck, but this was well defined. *Bacillinum C.* was ordered, and the whole thing disappeared within the month, and the little lady has been very thriving ever since.

So far as I am concerned in this work (*New Cure for Consumption*), the curability of ringworm by *Bacillinum* is an established fact and I therefore take leave of the subject so far as this work (*New Cure for Consumption*) is concerned.

Here in this little volume I am concerned purely with the question of ringworm from the organismic standpoint, and so I will adduce a little more clinical evidence from my case-book.

Neumann's statement that

healthy people are as liable to pityriasis versicolor and herpes tonsurans as those who are delicate I absolutely deny. Eczema marginatum is pretty common, and, therefore, I have seen a good many cases of it. Neumann is of opinion that eczema marginatum is a modified form of herpes tonsurans, which I doubt, as one meets with eczema marginatum in many fairly vigorous adult males, though they may not be truly *healthy*.

Moreover, eczema marginatum does not yield to *Bacillinum*. Eczema marginatum I have known to improve under the influence of this remedy, but that is all. If, therefore, eczema marginatum is the same thing mycologically as herpes tonsurans, there must be in its modification a *tertium quid*, a different pathological entity.

Four Cases of Ringworm (Sisters) cured by Internal Medication.

Miss Winnie X., aged ten, came under my care in the month of July 1891 to be treated for ringworm. There were several large patches on her scalp and numerous little ones; the largest was on the crown of the head, a trifle to the left, and nearly two inches in diameter. The child had a profuse mass of hair; is of fairly healthy parentage. I say fairly, because I formerly cured her mother of an abdominal tumour and her brother of very severe eczema. Winnie herself is small for her age, thin, and not robust looking, though she has been living in a fine healthy part of Yorkshire. Her neck was thin, and on both sides studded with feelable, large, hard glands. I put her on *Bacillinum* in my wonted way; in a month her glands were smaller and the herpes tonsurans was less active; and in three months the glands of her neck were well, she had grown, had taken on a healthy look—quite ruddy—and the ringworm was nearly gone, the hair all growing again. At the end of the fourth month she was in all respects normal, and a bright, bonny girl, and so she continues

The three other sisters of Winnie had the same disease, and the same general conditions of non-thriving; numerous pretty large, hard glands on both sides of the neck, and patches of the ringworm on their scalps and necks, and, like Winnie, with the bald ringworm patches, great shocks of hair. They had the same treatment for the same length of time, and with the identical result: the ringworm quite disappeared, the indurated glands got well (*i. e.*, impalpable), the girls took to growing, and took on a ruddy, healthy appearance. The cure of the ringworm in these four cases—as also in my others—was effected solely by the internal treatment by high potencies of *Bacillinum*. The improvement was gradual, general, and all along the line, as one, indeed, should theoretically expect from any remedial agent that cures organismically and organically. Note well; the cure is not only organismic, but *organic; not* chemical, *not* mechanical, *not* local, *not* topic, *not* antiparasitic, but organic, *vital.* The fungi are not attacked, but the "host" of the fungi is healed, and the wee fungi die, and their spores cannot germinate any further in the same soil. In these four cases three of them had profuse heads of hair hanging down their necks; one had been cropped. I ordered these fine heads of hair *not* to be cut off, but just left so as to put the treatment to the severest possible test, by thus leaving the spores of the fungi *en masse* all over the place. But this notwithstanding, no further development took place after the patients got well under the influence of the remedy, the progressive amelioration being steady, continuous, and complete. There are two elements in herpes tonsurans to be thus considered: *1st*, the soil-quality; and, *2nd*, the fungi. Every organic thing needs certain conditions of its own life in order to thrive, and what I maintain in regard to ringworm is, that the disease proper is not to be sought in the presence of the fungi, but in that quality of the body which constitutes its fitness for the fungi to develop and thrive. In other words, a really healthy individual does not, and cannot catch ringworm. I say *catch*, and by that I mean get it from ordinary together-living with ringwormy individuals. I do *not* refer to *inoculability*, where force is used, and the stuff is injected into one's flesh and blood direct, because here a new order of things is created, which fact is commonly entirely lost sight of. I will, however, not touch upon this question here, contenting myself with observing that *catching a complaint* in the common and natural order of things, and being *compelled* to take it by the injunction of material quantities of its stuff, are not equivalent by any means, though Pasteur, Koch, and biological experimenters very generally work and write as if they were. And this, indeed, constitutes the weak link in their chain of argument. More particularly is this the case with Koch and his experiments in tuberculosis. True, he renders certain (*healthy*) creatures by inoculations immune against tuberculosis, but our tubercular patients are not by any means healthy, but very unhealthy, inasmuch as they are tuberculous, and they can only be cured slowly, organically, by the processes set up by the action of homœopathic potencies of the remedy; for, if anything like a material dose be used, the action set up is on the same line and in the same direction as the disease, whereas the homœopathic high potency of the virus sets up a contrary—the opposite—action which tends to cure. This is the true reading of the phenomena, and this reading sheds light upon the whole subject, and affords a sound working hypothesis, and all the known phenomena are thus readily comprehended, and stand out in the clear light of reason tallying exactly with experience. Only the homœopathic law of the double and opposite action of different doses renders the use of viruses as remedies possible.

The greater the poison the greater the remedy; true, but only homœopathically. Throw out the homœopathic law, and the high potency and you are stranded, and your virus is a virus and nothing more; and where is Koch? Stranded just here—at this very point. He casts aside the homœopathic law, he ignores the possibility of the action of high potencies, and tries nevertheless to cure with likes or identicals, and he fails; and he not only fails to cure, but he kills, as do all who follow him, as he and their own published results clearly testify.

This is very unfortunate for sick folks, because the world at large do not, cannot, readily see the difference between the use of a virus in homœopathic potency and its use in Kochian fashion, ALTHOUGH THE RESULTS ARE EXACTLY OPPOSITE.

For them—medical and lay—tuberculinum is tuberculinum whether the matrix substance or a homœopathic potency, whereas the one is a poison that kills, while the other is a grand harmless remedy, that cures a very dire and fatal disease.

The vast majority of the homœopathic practitioners of the world take up this position: they say the use of viruses as remedies is not permissible; they are superior persons who disdain the use of such unspeakable things. They object to the kind of remedy altogether, which would be a tenable position if only they were able to cure as well without them. But can they? No, they cannot, and do not. I have before now urged, that inasmuch as the virus can (and must) be used in a high potency, what the origin or nature of the matrix may be is a matter of absolute indifference.

"Oh," say they, "but we do not believe in high potencies, there is nothing in them."

Their position is therefore this:

they object to, say, tuberculinum, or pyrogenium, because of their nature and origin; they object to them in high potency, because high potencies contain nothing at all. When, therefore, any of these superior persons object to the use of *Bacillinum* for the cure of ringworm on the ground of its being a virus, my reply is, that as I only use high potencies of it, and as high potencies, on their own showing, contain nothing at all, their objection falls to the ground, being reduced to the absurd, for no one can ascribe bad qualities to "nothing."

I will pass on now from the objections of these superior persons to a further study of the clinical results obtained by *Bacillinum* in the treatment of ringworm, and this I do the more willingly as I know full well that it were vain to expect or wait for any progress or help in the cure of grave forms of disease from them. They are now, therapeutically, where they formerly were, and in the future they will be still in the same place, subserving the not altogether useless purpose of milestones on the road of medical progress. They are already a good way behind, and will soon be lost to view altogether.

Homœopathy must progress on the lines of pathology and morbid anatomy, or it will wane, and study on animals will have to help us.

Case of Tinea Circinnata.

A young lassie of eight years of age was brought by her mother to me on February 18, 1889, for a patch of ringworm on the left side of the nose and several others on the back of the neck, where the hairy scalp ends. She had from me *Morbillinum* 30.

March 20.—The old spots have gone, but she has quite a number of new ones on chest and arms; her tongue is pippy; she does not get off to sleep very readily. There is no ringworm on the body.

℞ *Bacillinum C.*

This quite cured the ringworm, and it never returned. I should have stated at the outset of this little narration, that patient had

had ringworms for many months before she was brought to me at all.

Three years later—i. e., April 11, 1892—I again saw this girl with her mother, when I inquired whether there had been any return of the ringworm? Patient had almost forgotten all about the affair, but her mother exclaimed,—"Oh, Kathleen has never had any return of the ringworm, though fresh places had kept on coming for over a year when I first brought her to you."

Case of Ringworm Cured by Bacillinum CC.

Towards the end of the year 1891, a lady was induced by relatives to bring her twelve-year-old son to me, because he had suddenly arrived home from school with a circular, bald, scaly patch on the top of his head. The ring was about the size of a florin, and for the past three weeks had been treated most actively; one might say that said little ring-shaped patch had been attacked with venom, fury, and hatred by the surgeon, the mother, the governess, and by "uncle," the general impression conveyed by the onslaught was "we'll soon get rid of you!"

But in vain, though "uncle" is a general in the army. The indurated glands in the neck, the dusky colour of the skin of the neck, the dirt that would not wash off, showed quite clearly that the stroma was ill. Three months of the *Bacillinum CC.*, and nothing else locally or internally, effected a very perceptible change in the boy: not only had the nasty horror-inspiring ring-shaped patch become covered with clean, healthy hairs, but the scurf had gone, and the boy had grown an inch; he looked fresher, brighter, and—"Doctor, his face and neck are *so much* cleaner."

The boy duly returned to school in capital health.

Said the boy's mother, "I am beginning to have faith in your treatment, but oh! what a life 'uncle' and the others have led me."

What does your uncle say, now the nasty thing has gone?

"He says he always had his doubts as to whether it was a *true* case of ringworm."

But I thought he was so very sure about it?

"So he was when I brough S. to you, but the general says that the real ringworm is a parasitic disease, and that you cannot possibly kill parasites on the skin by giving the infected person little white powders to take."

Tell your uncle I think faith did it.

I fancy the general has a sure cure of his own brought from India.

Ringworm in General Survey in Literature.

In daily life we find ringworm a difficult disorder to cure: a few cases yield to almost any sensible treatment, but the bulk of them offer a stubborn resistance. And yet we often find the therapeutics of ringworm in the text-books confined to a very few lines. One author of no mean standing tells us that the soft-soap treatment generally suffices! However, some authors do not hesitate to speak out plainly on the subject. And I notice that the more the authors know of ringworm, the more they have studied it, the less therapeutically positive do they become. Willan (1817) confessed that it is "hard to cure."

Gruby (1844) made the discovery that a fungus was present in the broken-off hairs and in their root sheaths. This parasite was fully described by Malmsten, in Stockholm, in 1845, and it was named by him the Trichophyton tonsurans. Cazenave's name, Herpes tonsurans, is most commonly met with in many works. Its other names are legion.

Alder Smith, M. B. Lond., F. R. C. S. ("*Ringworm: Its Diagnosis and Treatment*," London 1885), has very usefully spent many years in studying ringworm, and in the work just named shows himself a thorough master of the subject, his position as Resident Medical Officer at Christ's Hospital, London, affording him incomparable opportunities for such studies. I shall take this author as the representative of the latest views of science on the subject of ringworm.

Alder Smith thus defines ringworm :—

"Ringworm is a disease of the skin caused by a microscopic vegetable parasite; and the characteristic lesions are due to this minute fungus invading the epithelial layers of the skin, the hair follicles, and the hairs. The growth which causes this very troublesome affection belongs to the lowest order of plant life, the fungi or moulds; the same fungus is found both in ringworm of the head and the body, and the two affections are essentially one. This disease, which is a very common one, is liable to attack all classes—the rich as well as the poor—and is highly contagious, but it is almost entirely confined to children." And then says:—

"The history of ringworm is

complicated, as certain varieties of form of the disease have received a number of designations from the older authors."*

As to the life-history of the fungus I will refer my readers to Alder Smith's work, which is beyond compare the best epitome of

* "*Viz.*—Porrigo scutullata, *Willan;* herpes tonsurans, herpes squamosus, *Cazenave;* herpes circinatus, *Bateman;* porrigo ton soria, dartre furfuracée arrondie, *Alibert;* tinea tondens, squarus tondens, *Mahon;* phyto-alopecia, *Malmstem;* rhizophyto-alopecia, trichophytie, *Gruby;* dermatomycosis tonsurans, *Köbner;* tinea trichophytina, tinea circinata, *Anderson;* trichonosis furfuracea; porrigo furfurans; lichen herpetiformis, *Devergie;* lichen circumscriptus, figuratus, gyratus, impetigo figerata, etc.; *Germ.*, scherende flechte; *Fr.*, herpes tonsurant; teigne tondante; teigne tonsurante."

the subject with which I am acquainted, almost all the other works on ringworm are antiquated and only of historic value. But I must quote what Alder Smith says of the *host* of the *Trichophyton tonsurans.*

"*The Soil.*"

"All children are not equally susceptible to ringworm. A certain unknown condition of the skin is necessary for the growth of the fungus, as some children never take ringworm though constantly liable to become infected For it is evident that when one child in a family has ringworm, and is not under any treatment, the others must be exposed to the action of the fungus; yet, at times, the disease does not spread.

"This fact is often used as an argument by parents, to prove that their children are not suffering from any contagious form of disease, and that they are in a fit condition to enter a school.

"On some the fungus takes but slight hold, and is easily destroyed. Others are extremely susceptible; the disease quickly attacks the follicles and the hairs, and spreads with great rapidity although under treatment. Sometimes treatment even accelerates the already rapid spread of the disease, by producing impetiginous eczema with crusts; and, by means of the pus, the fungus is carried to more distant and healthy parts. This variety is most difficult to manage.

"The difference in these cases

must depend on some peculiar nutritive condition of the soil or material in which the fungus develops, or upon some special state of the general health or constitution. In fact the state of the soil is a most important condition; and the rapidity with which a small spot of ringworm will spread before it comes under efficient treatment depends chiefly upon this peculiar condition of the soil or nidus. We generally find that ringworm specially occurs, and spreads most rapidly among poorly nourished children of a strumous or lymphatic diathesis.* And it is often

* "Mr. M. Morris states—and I fully agree with him—'that children with very light brown, golden, or colourless hair, with light grey or blue eyes, and with

observed that all the children in a family of this description, if they become infected, will suffer severely; evidently showing that there is some general condition present favouring the parasitic growth.

"Ringworm is also commonly seen amongst those who, while they are not decidedly strumous, are yet thin and pallid.

"Most children with *chronic* ringworm dislike fat; this avoidance of fat in the diet—according to Dr. Fox—'has a most potent influence in leading to the development of a condition of nutrition which is favourable to the occurrence of obstinate ringworm.'

fine skin with thin epidermis, take ringworm easily, and usually have it severely.'—*The Lancet*, Jan. 29th, 1881.

"But, on the other hand, we constantly see both recent and chronic ringworm in those who are neither strumous nor ill-nourished,—in fact upon decidedly healthy and robust children. This leads me still to hold the opinion, that the peculiar condition which is favourable to the development of the ringworm fungus is unknown.

"Ringworm does not exercise any noticable influence on the general organism or constitution, or on the general nutrition of the body."

I cannot agree with Dr. Fox's view, just quoted, in regard to the avoidance of fat as a food; what I would say is this: These children dislike fat because they are in an ill condition; the ill condition pre-exists the avoidance of fat, and is not produced by want of it, other than secondarily. Alder Smith, as we see, holds the opinion that "*we constantly see both recent and chronic ringworm* in those who are neither strumous nor ill-nourished—in fact, *upon decidedly healthy and robust children.*"

This I deny; the ringworm mould cannot grow on *really* healthy children any more than fish can live out of water. They may look healthy, even very healthy; they may appear to be robust, jolly, rosy, fat, but they are not truly healthy, or their skin-surface would not get mouldy in ringwormy patches.

Of course, my opportunities for observing ringworm are not by any means to be compared to those of

Alder Smith's, but I have examined a goodly number to test the point, and have never yet found a truly healthy child the subject of ringworm: they all have more or less indurated glands somewhere. From the curative results following the exhibition of *Bacillinum* I am led to believe that the mould of ringworm can only grow on those who are more or less strumous or tubercular, and that the degree of the disease gauges the degree of the constitutional morbidity.

Now Alder Smith is a reliable observer, a man of science and fact, and there is strong inherent evidence in his work on ringworm that he puts his facts fairly and squarely before his readers. This being so, it must follow that *his* facts should prove the constitutional nature of ringworm if such be the case.

Let us see.

ALDER SMITH'S FACTS VERSUS ALDER SMITH'S VIEW THAT "DECIDEDLY HEALTHY CHILDREN" MAY BE SUBJECT TO RINGWORM.

In the following quotations from Alder Smith's work most of *the italics are mine.*

He says (pp. 29 *et seq.*):—

"*Diagnosis of Ringworm which has Existed Some Time.*

"*Chronic Squamous Ringworm.*

"In the first place, I cannot help observing that very few medical men, either in consultation or private practice, are aware how *extremely difficult some cases of ring-*

worm are to cure; and the majority consider a case well, even when it has assumed a decidedly chronic state. I constantly have boys brought to me on their return to private schools, and very many also on their presentation for admission to Christ's Hospital, *who, while bringing certificates from medical men of the highest professional standing that they are cured of ringworm*, and quite fit to mix with other children, *are still suffering from a severe, contagious, and chronic form of the disease;* and I have often found on inquiry, that an opinion has been formed, and a certificate given without any special examination of the scalp, and certainly without the help of the lens or microscope. *Many practitioners imagine that ringworm is cured when some of the hair is again growing freely and firmly on the part affected.* This is a great mistake, as some of the most chronic and intractable cases are those in which the hair has partially grown again on the scurfy patches; but, on close inspection with a lens, *some short broken-off hair or stumps may be seen scattered among the healthy hairs.*

"It is impossible to speak too strongly on this point, as an outbreak of ringworm in a school is often due to the admission into it of an unrecognised case of the disease. As a rule, the trouble arises from a boy returning to school (after he has had an attack of ringworm on the head) *with a certificate to the effect that he is cured, when in fact he is suffering from a chronic and contagious form of the complaint;* or, from the entry into the school of an entirely unsuspected case; generally a boy, who has had a scurfy patch on his head for some time, but who is, in reality, suffering from chronic ringworm.

"Speaking from experience, after the examination of a very large number of children, both in private and for admission into Christ's Hospital and other schools, *I have found that in by far the majority of cases where a boy has had ringworm on the head within a year or two of my seeing him, the disease has not been really cured.* As a rule, the treatment has been continued until some new hair has made its appearance on the patches, after which it has been discontinued, although many diseased stumps remained. When this stage has been reached, *the case will often continue in the same chronic state*—the patches remained about the same size, *getting neither better nor worse*—while the little patient, who may be certified as "perfectly well," may be the constant and *unsuspected* cause of a succession of outbreaks of ringworm in a school."

We therefore see that in *by far the majority of cases* certified as cured the disease has not been cured at all, but still exists as *Chronic Squamous Ringworm.* Hence it follows that the ordinary statistics of the cure of ringworm by medical and surgical practitioners are worthless. The cures are not real, the treatment has merely got rid of the worst of the ringwormy mould in its more gross and evident form. Even one year, even two years, after the cure the sufferers continue to be contagiously ringwormy notwithstanding the fact that the patches have been scoured clean and the hairs have grown again.

Our Author further says:—

"*Disseminated Ringworm.*

"Especially would I call attention to a variety I call "disseminated ringworm"—*one rarely diagnosed*, and *the most chronic and difficult to cure*. The hair is found to be growing freely and firmly all over the head; there are, perhaps, no patches to be seen now, although probably they have existed at an earlies stage of the disease; the skin appears generally healthy, and perhaps almost free from scurf: but numerous isolated and generally thickened stumps, or groups of stumps, or black dots, are seen here and there, often scattered all over the scalp. *This variety is almost always overlooked*, and can only be detected by very careful examination."

And again:—

"*Diffuse Ringworm.*

"A very chronic form, "diffuse ringworm," is also sometimes seen, in which there are one or more large .irregular patches, often extending nearly all over the scalp.

The surface is very scurfy, and very many of the long hairs have grown again, but numerous stumps are to be seen in every direction. *This variety is constantly overlooked*, or mistaken for seborrhœa or chronic squamous eczema; but it can always be diagnosed by the stumps. Cases are even found where the entire scalp is affected.

"*Chronic Pustular Ringworm.*

"Chronic ringworm may also occur in the form of pustular spots, with a certain amount of redness and crusting around, and with a stump existing in the centre of each spot. This appears to be Nature's effort to get rid of the stump, and can be successfully imitated by treatment.

"*Small Spots.*

"Sometimes *chronic ringworm may exist*, *without apparent change*, *for months or even years*, as a single spot, or in spots so small that *they are not noticed*, even by professional men, with numerous long hairs and only a few stumps. Often ten minutes or more has to be spent in examining a child's head before any stumps can be detected. I have known an outbreak of ringworm in a school to be caused by a chronic spot *not larger than a split pea*, and where only a few stumps could be found on close examination with a lens."

We see, then, that not only are most of the cases certified by eminent medical men as cured, *not* really cured, but that "Disseminated Ringworm," "Diffuse Ringworm," and "Small-Spot Ringworm" are "rarely diagnosed," "constantly overlooked," and "not noticed even by professional men."

It must, therefore, be manifest that the germs of ringworm must be about in almost every gathering of children, at every party, in every school, in almost every church and chapel in the world; and when we further remember that Dr. Tilbury Fox found the conidia of trichophyton in abundance *in the dust deposited from the air* of a ward in which ringworm cases were located, it must be pretty clear that ringworm may be communicated through the air in a multitude of different places, and in almost all schools and other places where children do congregate, and that is practically everywhere. Alder Smith further affirms (p. 5) that it may be caught from the heads or infected articles belonging to boys or girls, with *chronic*, and often *unknown* and *untreated*, varieties of the disease, which are every day mistaken for chronic scruf or dry eczema.

Therefore we may say that the germs of ringworm are practically everywhere. This is quite what we should expect from our knowledge of the moulds generally: given the right conditions for mouldiness and moulds, and there they are. Also, given the right soil and conditions for ringworm—and there it is.

The other known facts of the

disease ringworm leads us to the same conclusion as just stated probable universal presence of the germs of ringworm.

Keeping still to our Author, we read (p. 44):—"I am positive that a ringworm on the head, the size of a sixpence, can develop in forty-eight hours, and increase to the size of a florin in another twenty-four hours, because I have actually seen ringworm grow at this rate. But this is certainly not the usual rate of progress. Ringworm generally develops much more slowly than this; yet there is no doubt that a moderate sized patch may appear in a few days.

"It cannot, on the other hand, be said how long it has not existed; for the place may spread very slowly, and remain almost in the same state for weeks, or even months.

"Cases like these (chronic ringworm) must have existed some time; probably for many months, *or possibly for years.*

"I remember one inveterate *case that resisted all treatment for nine years*, and though the patient was eighteen when I last saw him, *he still had disseminated ringworm; and another disseminated case* (*lately under my care*) *had been treated by many medical men for a period of eight years without being cured.*

"It is impossible to say how long even a small spot of chronic ringworm may not have existed, as *it may have remained in a latent state for month*, *or even years.*

"The rate of growth and rapidity

of reproduction are very different in individual cases. *If the fungus spreads slowly, it indicates only a slightly favourable soil,* and it can then—in its early stage—often be quickly eradicated; *but if it grows rapidly, it is due to the general nutritive condition furnishing a favourable nidus: it is then most difficult, and sometimes impossible to arrest its course; the increase in the rate of growth of the fungus being greater than can be counterbalanced by rubbing in parasiticides.*

"Dr. T. Fox says: 'Ringworm is *obstinate in proportion as this or that patient offers a favourable soil* in his textures for the growth of the fungus or parasite.'"

I think the impartial will at once concede that Alder Smith the physician completely refutes Alder Smith the rubber-in of parasiticides, but that he should do it unbeknown to himself is distinctly curious.

Is Ringworm a Disease Due to Dirt?

No; not one of my cases of the past three or four years was due to dirt, all being members of the higher and upper middle classes, who tub and scrub, perhaps, even too much.

On this point Alder Smith says: "It is a great mistake to think ringworm is due to dirt. Of course neglected children with dirty heads are more likely to be exposed to, and to take the disease; but it constantly occurs in children whose heads are kept perfectly clean, and where all proper care is taken. No matter what precautions are observed with regard to cleanliness, *some* of the other children in a school will commonly take ringworm if an untreated case is accidentally admitted into it, no matter from what class of society the pupils be obtained." Note the *some.*

Our Author continues:—"Children *under ten* years of age seem more prone to take the disease than those who are older; and it is *very rarely contracted after the age of thirteen*, and *hardly ever* seen on the head in adults. Again, infants are not often infected.

"About puberty, ringworm is more manageable, and generally—even when it has existed for years

—it tends to get well spontaneously soon after this period."

Now if the essence of the disease is the fungus, and the treatment is to be addressed to the killing of the fungi, why should the age of the individual host have anything to do with the parasite? And how is it that it gets well spontaneously after puberty?

Alder Smith devotes over a hundred pages to the treatment of ringworm—killing the fungi—and I will conclude this part of my subject with a few of *his* intercurrent remarks on the difficulties of the task. He says:—

"Nothing is easier to cure than a patch of ringworm situated on the body, but it is a very different matter when it exists on the hairy scalp. Then the treatment is, as a rule, most disappointing. *Quick cures are very rare*, and sure results are only to be obtained by thorough and long-continued employment of active remedies.

"It is necessary to keep in mind the important facts, that the fungus is the essential cause of the mischief; that it soon extends to the bottom of the hair-follicles; that its destruction is indispensable in order to cure the disease; that the great difficulty in curing ringworm is not to find parasiticides, but to get them to penetrate deeply into the hair-follicles, and thus come into contact with the fungus.

"Remedies act in two ways: first, by destroying the fungus—parasiticides, such as boracic acid, sulphurous acid, and the oleates of copper and mercury; others act by setting up inflammation, and even exudation about the follicles, and by this means cure the disease—as croton oil; but by far the majority combine both these properties, as acetic and carbolic acids, Goa powder, chrysarobin, nitrate of mercury, etc.

"It is very unwise to make a large sore place on the scalp, especially in recent ringworm, as the pustular variety may thus be set up; and strong preparations should never be used to young children.

"*Selection of a Treatment.*

"There are hundreds of different ways of treating ringworm of the head, and many 'never-failing' nostrums, which are warranted to cure the disease in a few days or weeks.

"The reason why so many things are said to cure ringworm is due to two causes: firstly, many cases are only ringworm of the body; secondly, numberless children are said to be well, when they still have ringworm in the most chronic form, and thus remedies are said to cure cases that have never been influenced for good by them. I have so often drawn attention to this fact that this may appear mere repetition, but considering the number of children constantly sent to me already certified as 'cured,' who have ringworm in a contagious form, it would appear that all that has been written on this subject has made but little impression on some medical men.

"*The plain truth is that there is not a single plan (except the use of strong caustics which will form scars) which can be relied on with absolute certainty to cure ringworm of the head.* The rapidity with which different cases, of apparently equal severity, yield to similar treatment varies greatly. Some go on unchecked for months, or even years, and may even spread under good treatment—while others rapidly get well."

The next hundred pages of Alder Smith's work are devoted to parasiticides and their modes of application to kill the fungi, and all this is by, perhaps, the greatest living authority on ringworm—always, *bien entendu*, from the outside surgeon's standpoint. The treatment of ringworm by orthodoxy thus requires horse-clipper, scrubbing-brush, and ointment-pot, and, to identify the sinful fungi, a microscope.

Date, 1892.

Finally, in the light of the foregoing facts, it must be manifest to any thoughtful practitioner that annular scalp mould or ringworm is to be regarded as a constitutional affair, and the treatment should be addressed to the host and not to the parasite.

We have seen that the germs of ringworm are almost universally present, and that at all times. The treatment by parasiticides is difficult, tedious, and, for the most part, entirely unsatisfactory, for the vast majority of cases medically certified as cured are really not cured at all.

The nephew of one of the best-known dermatologists of this country was lately brought by his mother to me to be treated for an ill-defined pining condition and a trifling cough. "He has never been well since he had the ringworm," exclaimed his mother. An examination of the boy's scalp showed that we had to do with pretty severe scalp eczema, or Alder Smith's Diffuse Chronic Ringworm. There was anorexia, and restless nights had brought down patient's state of nutrition. His cervical glands were hard and visible: two months of *Bacill.* and the boy was discharged well, or rather the mother did not bring him again, as he was in her judgment "perfectly well."

"But," said the mother, "I have come this time about myself; ever since my children had the ringworm last year my own head is covered with scurf, and my hair breaks off, and my hair has become quite thin and short, whereas I have always been so proud of my beautiful head of hair, especially as I have had so many children."

After being two months under the influence of *Bacillinum* in high potency and infrequently administered, the lady wrote to me saying, "my head is now quite free from scurf, and the hair is growing again beautifully." No external application of any kind soever was used; nor was any change made either in diet, mode of life, or place of abode.

Depend upon it, impartial reader, the mould of ringworm is not the disease; the disease is of the organism.

The Literature of Ringworm and of Mycology Generally.

Alder Smith I have quoted from largely, and his work, *Ringworm: Its Diagnosis and Treatment*, third edition, London, 1885, is classic.

Then there is Cooke's *Fungi: Their Nature, Influence, and Uses*, which is a masterly production.

Besides these I have also consulted the following from my own library, viz.:—

1. *Mushroom-Culture for Amateurs*, by W. J. May.
2. *British Fungi*, by E. M. Holmes, F. L. S., F. R. M. S. London, 1886.
3. *Parasitic Diseases of the Skin, Vegetoid and Animal*, by James Startin. London, 1881.
4. *A Synopsis of the Bacteria and Yeast Fungi*, by W. B. Grove, B. A. London, 1884.
5. *Micro-Fungi*, by Thomas Brittain. Manchester, 1882.
6. *The Plant-World: Its Past, Present, and Future*, by George Massee. London, 1891.
7. *Rust, Smut, Mildew, and Mould: An Introduction to the Study of Microscopic Fungi*, by M. C. Cooke, M. A., LL. D., A. L. S. London, 1886.

8. *An Essay on Ringworm*, by Andrew Paul, surgeon, Oxford, 1849.

9. *Les Microbes Pathogènes*, par Ch. Bouchard, Membre de l'Institut, Paris, 1892.

10. *On Ringworm: An Inquiry into the Pathology, Causes, and Treatment*, by William J. Smith, M. B. Lond. London, 1867.

11. *On Ringworm: Its Causes, Pathology, and Treatment*, by Erasmus Wilson, F.R.S. London, 1847.

But I had not by any means the wish to write the history of my subject; I merely desired to get a look round in the literature of the subject generally: only an all-round idea leading up to the study of pathogenous fungi.

Ringworm Regarded from the Standpoint of General Mycology.

The botany of most medical men can be at best only a of very elementary nature, and when we come to a consideration of the physiology of the fungi this is especially so. To have independent views of mycological questions from the standpoint of botanic science I should need a vast deal more knowledge of fungi than I can claim; but at the same time I am anxious to see whether my clinical standpoint is at variance or in consonance with the views of acknowledged mycologists. For it must be manifest that we might expect to find certain fixed data in the physiology of fungi generally that should help us somewhat in arriving at a just conclusion.

Cooke* almost doubts the possibility of excluding the germs of common fungi, so numerous are they, and no air can be found but what contains multitudes of them.

According to Pasteur the spores of fungi are more numerous near human habitations.

A very common form of mould is *Penicillium*, its spores being everywhere present in large numbers.

* *Fungi: Their Nature, Influence, and Uses*, by M. C. Cooke, M.A., LL.D., etc. London, 1875.

Neumann* says that the results of his experiments confirm the clinical observation of Hebra as to the origin of Herpes tonsurans (ringworm) and favus from one organism, viz., *Penicillium.*

Hallier regards *Trichophyton* as a development of the conidia chains of *Penicillium.* It must, therefore, be manifest that any one may have ringworm without ever coming into contact with ringworm as such at all, inasmuch as the conidia of *Penicillium* are the germs of *Trichophyton*, and the conidia of *Penicillium* are always present in large

* *Text book of Skin Diseases*, by Dr. Isidor Neumann, Lecturer on Dermatology in the Imperial University of Vienna. Translated by Dr. Pullar. London, 1871.

quantities in the atmospheric air wherein we live, and move, and have our being. And hence it would appear that the presence or absence of ringwormy boys in a school is not a matter of capital importance, inasmuch as the ringworm mould is only another and higher form of the *Penicillium*.

There is so much evidence on record illustrating the polymorphism of fungi, that it cannot be regarded as a very far cry from *Penicillium* to *Trichophyton*.

Grove* speaks with small respect of the reliability of the data given by medical mycologists. His di-

* *A Synopsis of the Bacteria and Yeast Fungi and Allied Species* (*Schizomycetes and Saccharomycetes*), by W. B. Grove, B.A. London, 1884.

vision of fungi into chromogenous, zymogenous, and pathogenous seems fairly natural.

Speaking of fungi, Holmes* says:—"Mushrooms, toadstools, the mildew on walls, the mould on bread, the rust on wheat, and the potato disease, are familiar objects to most of us; but few who are not botanists are aware that they all belong to the large and varied group of plants comprised under the name of fungi. It might be still more surprising to some to learn that the yeast with which bread is made and beer fermented, the vinegar plant which is used to turn sugar and water into vinegar,

* *British Fungi, Lichens and Mosses, including Scale-Mosses and Liverworts*, by E. M. Holmes, F.L.S., etc. London, 1886.

and the disagreeble skin disease called ringworm, all belong to the same class of plants."

He also tells us that many species which in this country are despised as loathsome toadstools, form regular articles of diet in Italy, Russia, and other countries; while in China and Japan several kinds of fungi are cultivated on decaying trunks of trees, in the same way that mushrooms are grown in the catacombs of Paris. Not very pleasant for one enjoying a *petit diner* in a beautiful Parisian café to suddenly remember that the daintly dressed mushrooms in the dish before him were perhaps grown in the catacombs.

The role played by the fungi in this world of ours almost baffles any adequate conception ; to them we owe beer, wine, vinegar, our very bread (in the form we use it), and—ringworm.

Concluding Thoughts.

X. the organic individual dies, and as spores and germs are everywhere present, they find in the decaying X. their food, housing, and all their other conditious of organic and organismic thrift. The death of X. is birth to innumerable organisms, for as soon as X. ceases to react with its medium, then these organisms begin their life on its organic remains. Life is just change. Nature knows no dead material, for the grave of one organism is the birthplace of many more; the animal lives on the vegetal, and man lives on them both. *En revanche* man decays and dies, and vegetal and animal again swarm into being in his remains. Verily, an awful contemplation, but so it indubitably is. Then there is another death in the form of emanations; our very breath is death in a certain sense. The products of any assembly of organisms at a given stage of intensity poison and kill their producers, they getting diseases constituting their ante-mortal stage. It is just the same throughout Nature and with all degenera and species.

It is the degree of concentration that is really determinative.

The Hollyhock Disease.

Cooke (*jam cit.*) remarks that a

writer in the *Gardener's Chronicle* has proposed a remedy for the hollyhock disease which he hopes will prove effectual. He says:—"The terrible disease has now, for twelve months, threatened the complete annihilation of the glorious family of hollyhock, and to baffle all the antidotes that the ingenuity of man could suggest, so rapidly does it spread and accomplish its deadly work. Of this I have had very good evidence, as last year at this time I had charge of [the italics are mine], if not the largest, *one of the largest and* finest collections of *hollyhocks anywhere in cultivation*, which had been under my special care *for eleven years*, and up to within a month of my resigning that position I had observed nothing uncommon amongst them; but before taking my final leave of them, I had to witness the melancholy spectacle of *bed after bed* being smitten down, and amongst them many splendid seedlings which had cost me *years of patience* and anxiety to produce. And, again, upon taking a share and the management of this business, another infected *collection* fell to my lot, so that I have been doing cruel battle with this disease since its first appearance amongst us, and I must confess that up to a very short time back I had come in for a great deal the worst of the fight, although I had made use of every agent I could imagine as being likely to aid me, and all that many competent friends could suggest. But lately I was reminded of Condy's patent fluid, diluted with water, and at once produced a bottle of the green quality, and applied it in the proportion of a large tablespoonful to one quart of water; and upon examining the plants dressed, twelve hours afterwards, was delighted to find it had effectually destroyed the disease." And so on.

He continues:—"I believe planting the hollyhocks *in large crowded beds* should be *avoided*, as I have observed the *closer they are growing* the more virulently does the disease attack them, *whereas isolated rows* and plants are but *little injured*." Now the point brough out by this gardener with regard to his beautiful hollyhocks is precisely what my own ideas lead up to, viz., *overcrowding*. Let us note that our friend's hollyhocks were *in large numbers*, they had been *there a long time*, the *closer* they were growing the more virulently did the disease attack them, whereas isolated rows and plants were but little injured.

The lately prevailing epidemic of influenza is, in my judgment, a fungal disease produced *in houses*—*i. e.*, overcrowding.

During this epidemic I noticed that *house-life* was seemingly necessary for it to thrive. In one town the mortality was fearful, over 60 per 1000; it was difficult to get undertakers enough to bury the dead. I recommended my patients there to keep their windows wide open night and day, and where this was done *no one fell ill!*

The emanations of organisms, whether hollyhock or human beings, are of the nature of effete, dead matter, notably to the selfsame organisms, and, give a sufficient degree of concentration, fungal disease is the result. The Condy's fluid probably killed the hollyhock disease by using-up the autoinfective hollyhock emanations on which the fungi lived and throve; it would act in two ways, viz., by using-up the hollyhock emanations the hollyhocks had a poison-free medium again, and the fungi would become weak from want, and thus be readily killed, or simply die off wholesale from starvation.

We call to mind that the disease did not attack those hollyhocks that were isolated in single rows, their emanations not being here sufficiently concentrated to give the fungi enough to live on. We note well that the collection of hollyhocks, in which the disease became formidable, was *very large*, and had been long established in the same place.

The emanation of organisms are noxious and obnoxious to the self-same organisms. Any one can notice that where horses and cows graze in the same meadow the horses will nibble off the grass close to cow-dung but not near their own, and conversely the cows will eat the grass close to horse-dung, and even push it away with their mouths without evincing the slighest objection.

All creatures abhor their own dejecta. Even the "dirty pig" is *very* sty-clean if he has the chance, and evidently on the same principle, while he has no objection whatever to the dejecta of other animals.

Physicians know but too well the smells of bedrooms, and even a very large bedroom with only one healthy person in it for a very short time will get quite "frowsy" in an hour, particularly if the person has been to sleep.

The emanations from living organisms are very evidently hurtful to themselves, and, if sufficiently concentrated, more or less deadly, and it seems probable that the fungi come in and thrive thereon to the advantage of the organisms, tending at any rate to postpone the fatal issue; organic remains and emanations constitute the pabulum of the fungi. Of course the fungi must follow the ordinary law of Nature, and they in their turn must succumb to their own products.

Nature does not tolerate any dead thing, for as soon as there is any dead thing present new life starts therein forthwith. How far fungal products poison the hosts of the fungi is worthy of study and thought, and will in the future loom large into therapeutics.

It seems to me that those children who are suffering from ringworm are in better health with their ringworm than they are when the ringworm fungi are killed off by local measures. My own observations on this part of the subject are as yet too few for me to be able to form a positive opinion, but as far as they do go they tend to the conclusion that serious ill-health often dates from the time when they were *cured* of ringworm, *i.e.*, from the time when the fungi were locally more or less destroyed from the surface. I know of two cases in which very severe forms of deafness started coincidently with the germicidal cure of ringworm.

The thought naturally at once arises in one's mind, whether the trichophyton of ringworm has any relationship to the bacillus of tuberculosis, and if so, what?

Just as the fungal disease of hollyhocks was most virulent where they were crowded, so is the fungal disease ringworm in most evil report in *schools*, or, in other words, where the children are numerous and close together. Schoolmasters and school-surgeons are very positive about ringworm having been "imported into the school" by a boy coming from his home, but my own experience goes to show that as a rule ringworm is bred in the schools and is exported thence into the families. Not only so, but it is large families that supply us with specimens of ringwormy children more frequently than small ones, and it is the large schools that suffer most. At least so it appears to me from my only moderately numerous observations.

And in regard to tuberculosis we find this behaves similarly, and it is certainly true that where numerous human beings house together in closed apartments, there anthropotoxine* is generated, and the bacillus of tuberculosis finds its cradle and home. Of course, some organisms can withstand the effects of poisons, simply by reason of their strength, more than others; the weaker and more delicate deteriorate in health from the effects of anthropotoxine.

Anthropotoxine is inhaled until the lungs become bad enough for the fungus of phthisis to thrive in. I do not imagine that overcrowding acts in any specific way, or that

*The poisonous principle in human emanations.

numbers are necessary other than in proportion to the quantity of air to be breathed. It therefore follows that a household of two persons may suffer from overcrowding, while one of twenty persons may not,—it is the proportion; and always must we remember that there are several factors in the sum, viz., the lack of sufficient clean fresh air; the presence of autotoxine (the hollyhock emanations from the hollyhocks, and the anthropotoxine for human beings), and then fungal life. And then, given these forests of fungi, their effects upon their hosts have to be considered. This is a large chapter. Certainly fungi love darkness rather than light, but whether their deeds are therefore evil, science, experience, and thinking must determine.

Bland Sutton in his *Evolution and Disease* (London, 1890), and after a consideration of actinomycosis, a very interesting disease, expresses the view that sarcoma is of fungal nature, and as what he says on the subject is eminently instructive and intensely interesting, I cannot refrain from giving his summary :—

"To put the matter in a clear form, a sarcoma is probably the scene of action of a virulent and prolonged conflict between irritant micro-organisms and leucocytes. I say probably, because, as has been already remarked, bacteriologists have not yet succeeded in isolating a special bacterium for sarcomata in general; that such agents will soon be discovered is in the highest degree probable, because in recent years each increase in the list of infective granulomata is made at the expense of sarcomata. The structure, mode of growth, infective properties, and manner in which these tumours destroy life, clearly coincide with what is positively known with regard to infective granulomata. The fact that sarcomata make up the greater part of tumours occurring in wild and domesticated animals has, in my opinion, a very significant import in this relation."

Thus we see that although ringworm may not at first sight appear to offer a very promising subject of general interest, we soon find ourselves in studying it landed right into the middle of the great bio-pathological problem of "the maggot and the cheese"—*i. e.*, life and death.

It has been urged against some of the medical views to which I have given expression that they are advanced too positively as absolute facts; well, of course, that may be: I give my data and my reasons, so that any other competent medical person can judge for himself whether I am right or wrong. It is perfectly true that I am a positive individual; I believe in work and progress, and, in the practical activities of the physician, I want helpful, and, therefore, positive views. If I have bad ringworm cases to cure what is the use to me of the medical agnosticism of the superior person whose position is this:—

"It may be so, I cannot tell, and wouldn't like to say,
I don't incline to this or that, nor yet the other way;
I can't at any time feel sure, yet hardly like to doubt,
And feel I musn't trust to 'guess' for fear of being out
Not feeling any certainty, I do not like to speak,
I don't know what I want to know nor what I ought to seek
I never like to venture far for fear of running wide,
And I haven't any notion how I ever can decide."

Of ringworm I hold positively,—(1.) That it is a constitutional complaint. (2.) That it is generated by the together-being of numbers of young people in close spaces *i. e.*, by their personal emanations, or anthropotoxine. (3.) That it is so to speak, "subtuberculosis." (4.) That it is curable by its pathologic *simillimum*, here termed *Bacillinum*, in high potency, internally and infrequently administered. (5.) That the mycosis is merely the concomitant external manifestation of the disease and not the disease itself. (6.) That the external treatment of the disease is irrational, unscientific, and, probably, harmful to the patient. (7.) That it is commonly bred in schools. (8.) That truly healthy children cannot catch it because the fungus cannot grow upon such. (9.) There is, therefore, no reason why a ringwormy child should be excluded from school life or the company of its fellows in home life (10.) And, finally, that the trichophyton of ringworm is to ringworm what the bacillus of Koch is to tuberculosis,—the trichophyton and the bacillus being, moreover, nearly related to one another.

INDEX.

Agnosticism in medicine, 117.
Anthropotoxine, 113, 118.
Bacillic virus, 13, 15.
Bacillinum, 17, 18, 24, 27, 28, 36, 37, 38, 39, 41, 42, 50, 52, 53, 54, 67, 91.
Bacillus of tuberculosis, 111, 113, 119.
Burnett, Dr. J. C., Diseases of the Skin from the Organismic Standpoint, 3, 27.
Burnett, Dr. J. C., Five Years' Experience in the New Cure of Consumption by its own Virus, 11, 37.
Cases reported, 12, 13, 14, 22, 37, 40, 52, 53, 80, 90.
Cattle affected by ringworm, 31.
Concluding thoughts, 101.
Condy's patent fluid, 105, 107.
Consumption, Five Years' Experience in the New Cure of, by its own Virus, 11, 37.
Consumption, virus of, 11; influence of, on teeth, 12; on ringworm, 12, 14.

Cooke's, Dr. M. C., Fungi: their Nature, Influence, and Uses, 92, 96.

Cooke, Dr. M. C., on the hollyhock disease, 102.

Eczema marginatum, 38, 39.

Fox, Dr. Tilbury, on avoidance of fat in diet, 64.

Fox, Dr. Tilbury, on conidia of trichophyton, 77.

Fox, Dr. Tilbury, on obstinacy of ringworm, 81.

Gardener's Chronicle, writer in, 103.

Grove, W. B., Bacteria and Yeast Fungi, 98.

Gruby's discovery of fungus, 57.

Hallier on trichophyton and penicillium, 97.

Herpes circinnatus (ringworm of the surface) treated by sepia, 10.

Herpes s. tinea tonsurans (ringworm), 7.

Herpes tonsurans, 58, 97.

Hollyhock disease, the, 102.

Holmes, E. M., British Fungi, etc., 99.

Hughes' Manual of Therapeutics, 10, 11.

Köbner inoculated ringworm, 29.
Koch stranded, 47.
Malmsten, in Stockholm, describes parasite Trichophyton tonsurans, 57.
Medicine, agnosticism in, 117.
Morbillinum, 52.
Morris, M., on ringworm, 63.
Mycology, literature of, generally, 92.
Mycology, standpoint as regards ringworm, 95.
Neumann on ringworm and eczema marginatum, 38.
Neumann, results of his experiments, 97.
Pasteur on spores of fungi, 96.
Penicillium, 96, 97.
Pityriasis versicolor, 39.
Psora of the Homœopaths, 9.
Ringworm a constitutional complaint, 118.
Ringworm a fairly common complaint, 17.
Ringworm an external disease due to an external infection, the trichophyton, 29, 118.

Ringworm an internal disease of the organism, 21.
Ringworm as studied by Alder Smith, M. B., 58–89.
Ringworm, cases of, 12, 13, 14, 22, 37, 40, 52, 53, 80, 90.
Ringworm caught from cows, 36.
Ringworm, concluding thoughts on, 101.
Ringworm cured by Bacillinum, 17, 18, 24, 27, 28, 36, 37, 38, 42, 54, 118.
Ringworm, Dr. Tilbury Fox on, 64, 77, 81.
Ringworm due to a specific fungus, 7.
Ringworm, healthy children do not catch, 5, 44, 119.
Ringworm (Herpes s. tinea tonsurans), 7.
Ringworm in cattle, 31.
Ringworm in general survey in literature, 56.
Ringworm inoculated by Köbner, 29.
Ringworm, is it due to dirt? 82.
Ringworm is parasitic, 19, 119.
Ringworm, literature of, and of mycology, generally, 92, 118.

Ringworm of the surface (Herpes circinnatus)treated by sepia and tellurium, 10.

Ringworm, proper, of the scalp, treated by sepia or sulphurous acid, 11.

Ringworm regarded from the standpoint of general mycology, 92.

Ringworm, selection of a treatment for, 86.

Ringworm, treatment of, by external means, unsatisfactory, 20.

Sepia in Herpes circinnatus, 10.

Sepia in ringworm proper of the scalp, 11, 19, 27.

Skin, Diseases of the, from the Organismic Standpoint, 3. 27.

Smith, Alder, M. B., chronic pustular ringworm, 75.

Smith, Alder, M. B., diagnosis of ringworm which has existed some time, 68.

Smith, Alder, M. B., diffuse ringworm, 74, 90.

Smith, Alder, M. B., disseminated ringworm, 73.
Smith, Alder, M. B., on heads or infected articles, 78.
Smith, Alder, M. B., on ringworm, 58–89.
Smith, Alder, M. B., small spots, 76.
Sulphur, 19, 27.
Sulphurous acid in ringworm proper of the scalp, 11.
Sutton, Bland, Evolution and Disease, 115.
Tellurium in treatment of Herpes circinatus, 10, 19, 27.
Tinea circinata 52.
Tongue, yellow-coated, 4.
Trichophyton, 29, 97, 98, 111, 119.
Virus of consumption, 11, 13.
Willan on ringworm, 57.